THE MASTER-WORD IN MEDICINE

William Osler's

THE MASTER-WORD IN MEDICINE

A Study in Rhetoric

By

CHARLES G. ROLAND, M.D.

Chairman
Department of Biomedical Communications
Mayo Foundation
Associate Professor, History of Medicine
Mayo Graduate School

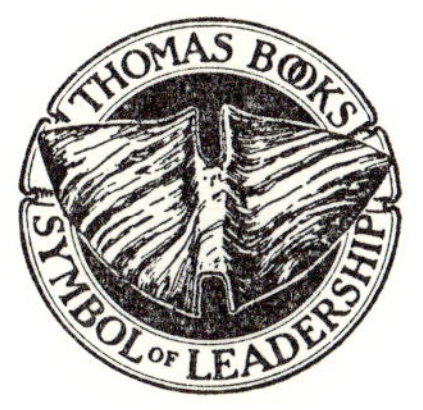

CHARLES C THOMAS · PUBLISHER
Springfield · Illinois · U.S.A

Published and Distributed Throughout the World by

CHARLES C THOMAS · PUBLISHER

BANNERSTONE HOUSE

301–327 East Lawrence Avenue, Springfield, Illinois, U.S.A.

NATCHEZ PLANTATION HOUSE

735 North Atlantic Boulevard, Fort Lauderdale, Florida, U.S.A.

© *1972, by* CHARLES C THOMAS · PUBLISHER

ISBN 0–398–02393–X

Library of Congress Catalog Card Number: 75–187673

With THOMAS BOOKS *careful attention is given to all details of manufacturing and design. It is the Publisher's desire to present books that are satisfactory as to their physical qualities and artistic possibilities and appropriate for their particular use. THOMAS BOOKS will be true to those laws of quality that assure a good name and good will.*

Printed in the United States of America

K-8

To Jay

INTRODUCTION

*T*he message that William Osler (1849–1919) brought to the students at the University of Toronto in 1903 was simple and timeless. I feel no need to apologize for reproducing that message, because students—and as Osler so rightly said, we are *all* students—can benefit from it in 1972 at least as well as in 1903.

Although I believe that there can be no argument with the message, the same cannot perhaps be said of the medium. Osler's language, and especially his rhetorical style, are those of seven decades ago. Why, you might ask, not simply present his message in the style of our day?

First, although the style may be somewhat dated, Osler's essay contains no serious obscurities. One can understand it well without having to translate it as one must translate Middle English; nor does it present complexities of syntax such as challenge readers of the prose of Sir Thomas Browne. So I do not believe I ask too much, when I present *The Master-Word in Medicine* to today's reader.

Secondly, there may be some merit in unusualness itself. Sometimes readers will pay more attention to a message just because it comes to them in a slightly different form, using a literary technique that is obviously old but not thereby invalid.

Further, there is more to Osler's message than his message. There is Osler himself. I am no idolater of the man but I have been infected with the magic of his personality, even though I know it no more than second and third hand. I believe that his benignly humanistic attitude, stressing the supremacy of sheer good manners and good taste in dealing with one's fellowman—whether patient, colleague, acquaintance, or passing stranger—urgently needs copying in our time. The attitude can only be taught by example, and examples are too few these days; next in value to his living example is some study of the writings of Osler. *The Master-Word in Medicine* reveals much of this most human and humane man.

Of Osler's many addresses, several were frankly and almost entirely inspirational in intent. In addition to *The Master-Word in Medicine*, there was *A Way of Life, Aequanimitas, Man's Redemption of Man,* and *Science and Immortality. The Master-Word in Medicine* was the second published of these five, appearing almost contemporaneously in six journals, including the *Montreal Medical Journal* and the *British Medical Journal,* in 1903, and again in the *Bulletin of the Johns Hopkins Hospital* in 1904.

In studying the *Master-Word,* it is important to keep in mind that it was an address. Some of its weaknesses as an essay would not have been apparent to those who heard Osler deliver it, and indeed at least one who attended the Toronto festivities has related how Osler achieved a real atmosphere of tension through the prolonged introduction to his *Master-Word.*

Cushing claims that this was one of Osler's more "finished" addresses. Certainly, it is typical Oslerian rhetoric. Three characteristics can be said to identify his speeches and writings: common sense, literary allusion, and reference to medical colleagues living and dead. The *Master-Word* abounds in all three.

The common sense I shall leave the reader the pleasure and profit of discovering for himself. It is to the other two elements that I have devoted my efforts in annotating the essay. But I hasten to say that the particular items I have chosen to describe do not comprise all the possibilities. Far from it. In some sentences the language sounds as if it derives from an earlier writer, but my scholarship is too scanty to identify the source. I have tried to elucidate every reference to which an author's name is attached, but I have not succeeded completely there either. The biographical allusions were less difficult to gloss, although I have not attempted to provide more than minimal identification.

Osler needs little introduction, and I fear I have been overlong. Let me give him the floor, taking further space only to quote Harvey Cushing's judgment of *The Master-Word in Medicine:* "Any student incapable of being uplifted by an exhortation of this kind is beyond the pale."

CHARLES G. ROLAND

THE MASTER-WORD IN MEDICINE

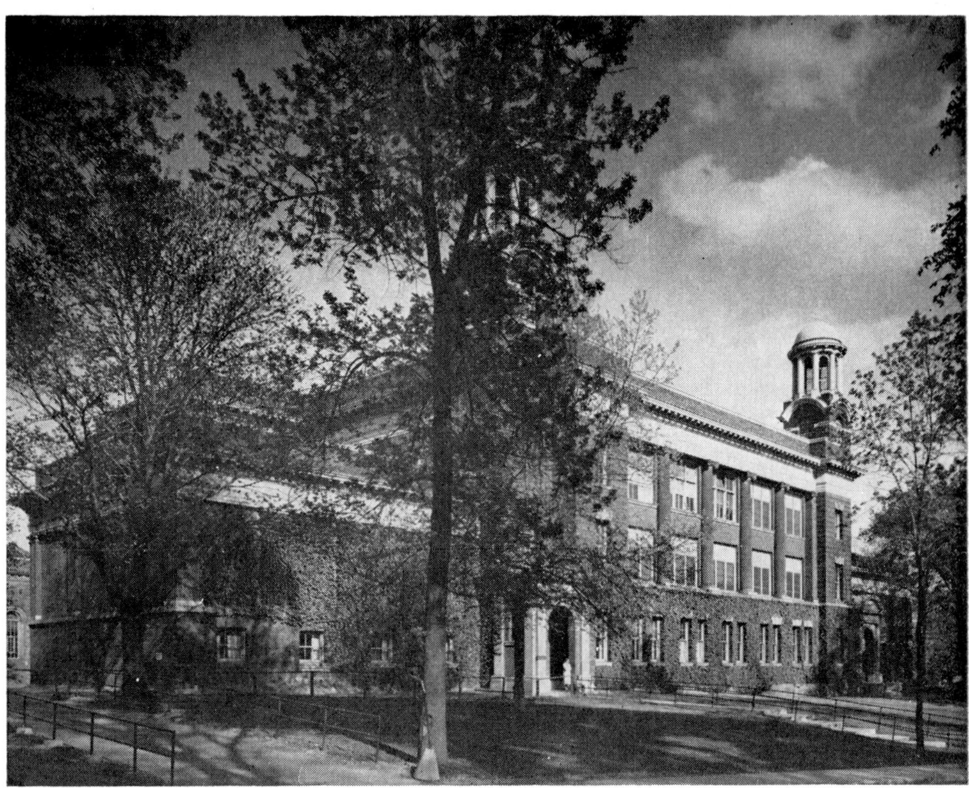

This was the building Osler helped to dedicate in 1903. It was demolished in 1968; in this building, in 1921, Banting and Best discovered insulin. (Courtesy of Department of Information, University of Toronto.)

I

$\mathcal{B}$efore proceeding to the pleasing duty of addressing the undergraduates, as a native of this province and as an old student of this school, I must say a few words on the momentous changes inaugurated with this session, the most important, perhaps, which have taken place in the history of the profession in Ontario. The splendid laboratories,[1] which we saw opened this afternoon, a witness to the appreciation by the authorities of the needs of science in medicine, make possible the highest standards of education in the subjects upon which our Art is based. They may do more. A liberal policy, with a due regard to the truth that the greatness of a school lies in brains, not bricks, should build up a great scientific center which will bring renown to this city and to our country. The men in charge of the departments are of the right stamp. See to it that you treat them in the right way by giving skilled assistance enough to ensure that the vitality of men who could work for the world is not sapped by the routine of teaching. One regret will, I know, be in the minds of many of my younger hearers. The removal of the departments of anatomy

1. See photograph on facing page.

and physiology from the biological laboratory of the university breaks a connection which has had an important influence on medicine in this city. To Professor Ramsay Wright[2] is due much of the inspiration which has made possible these fine new laboratories. For years he has encouraged in every way the cultivation of the scientific branches of medicine, and has unselfishly devoted much time to promoting the best interests of the Medical Faculty. And in passing let me pay a tribute to the ability and zeal with which Dr. A. B. Macallum[3] has won for himself a world-wide reputation by intricate studies which have carried the name of this University to every nook and corner of the globe where the science of physiology is cultivated. How much you owe to him in connection with the new buildings I need scarcely mention to this audience.

But the other event which we celebrate is of much greater importance. When the money is forthcoming, it is an easy matter to join stone to stone in a stately edifice, but it is hard to find the market in which to buy the precious cement which can unite into an harmonious body the professors of medicine of two rival medical schools in the same city.[4] That this has been accomplished so satisfactorily is a tribute to the good sense of the leaders of the two faculties, and tells of their recognition of the needs of the profes-

2. Ramsay Wright (1852–1933) was the first Professor of Biology at the University of Toronto. From 1901 till he retired in 1912 he was also Vice-President of the University and Dean of the Faculty of Arts. In 1887 Wright and A. B. Macallum reported on a new trematode, Sphyranura osleri (given "the specific name Osleri, in compliment to the original discoverer": J Morphol 1:1–48, 1887).

3. Archibald B. Macallum (1858–1934) was, when this essay was delivered, Professor of Physiology at the University of Toronto; apparently he was the first person in Canada to devote himself exclusively to research in basic science and to the teaching of that science. He was also the first Chairman of the National Research Council of Canada.

4. The Faculty of Medicine of the University of Toronto and the Medical Faculty of Trinity University, also in Toronto.

sion of the province. Is it too much to look forward to the absorption or affiliation of the Kingston and London schools into the Provincial University? The day has passed in which the small school without full endowment can live a life beneficial to the students, to the profession, or to the public. I know well of the sacrifice of time and money which is freely made by the teachers of those schools; and they will not misunderstand my motives when I urge them to commit suicide, at least so far as to change their organizations into clinical schools in affiliation with the central university as part, perhaps, of a widespread affiliation of the hospitals of the province. A school of the first rank in the world, such as this must become, should have ample clinical facilities under its own control. It is as much a necessity that the professors of medicine and surgery, etc., should have large hospital services under their control throughout the year, as it is that professors of pathology and physiology should have laboratories such as those in which we here meet. It should be an easy matter to arrange between the provincial authorities and the trustees of the Toronto General Hospital to replace the present antiquated system of multiple small services by modern well-equipped clinics—three in medicine and three in surgery to begin with. The increased efficiency of the service would be a substantial *quid pro quo,* but there would have to be a self-denying ordinance on the part of many of the attending physicians. With the large number of students in the combined school, no one hospital can furnish in practical medicine, surgery and the specialties a training in the art an equivalent of that which the student will have in the sciences in the new laboratories. An affiliation should be sought with every other hospital in the city and province of fifty beds and over, in each of which two or three extra-mural teachers could be recognized who would receive for three or more months a number of students proportionate to the beds in the hospital. I need not mention names. We all know men in Ottawa, Kingston, London, Hamilton, Guelph and Chatham, who could take charge of small groups of the senior students and make of them good practical doctors. I merely throw out the suggestion. There are difficulties in the way; but is there anything in this life worth struggling for which does not bristle with them?

Students of medicine: may this day be to each one of you, as it was to me when I entered this school thirty-five years ago, the beginning of a happy life in a happy calling. Not one of you has come here with such a feeling of relief as that which I experienced at an escape from conic sections and logarithms and from Hooker and Pearson. The dry bones became clothed with interest, and I felt that I had at last got to work. Of the greater advantages with which you start I shall not speak. Why waste words on what you cannot understand. To those only of us who taught and studied in the dingy old building which stood near here is it given to feel the change which the years have wrought—a change which my old teachers, whom I see here to-day —Dr Richardson,[5] Dr. Ogden,[6] Dr. Thorburn[7] and Dr. Oldright[8]—must find hard to realize. One looks about in vain for some accustomed object on which to rest the eye in its backward glance— all, all are gone; the old familiar places. Even the landscape has altered, and the sense of loneliness and regret, the sort of homesickness one experiences on such occasions, is relieved by a feeling of thankfulness that at least some of the old familiar faces have been spared to see this day. To me at least the memory of those happy days is a perpetual benediction, and I look back upon the two years I spent at this school with the greatest delight. There were many things that might have been improved—and we can say the same of every medical school at that period—but I seem to have gotten more out of it than our distinguished philosopher friend, J. Beattie Crozier,[9] whose picture of the period seems rather hardly drawn. But after all, as some one has remarked, instruction is often

5. James Henry Richardson (1823–1910) had the distinction of being the first graduate in medicine at the University of Toronto. Soon after, he became Professor of Anatomy, serving from 1850 until 1902, and was Surgeon to the Toronto Jail from 1859 until 1909.

6. Uzziel Ogden (1828–1910) taught, during his career, physiology, materia medica, and midwifery and gynecology; from 1880 till 1892 he was Dean of the Faculty of Medicine of Victoria College.

7. James Thorburn (1830–1905) taught pharmacology and therapeutics at the University of Toronto; in 1895 he was President of the Canadian Medical Association. According to his obituary he was "a staunch Liberal of the old school."

8. William Oldright (1842–1917) was born in the West Indies and died in Chicago, but spent most of his life in Toronto. A chief interest was hygiene, a subject that he taught at the University of Toronto; in 1882 he was the first Chairman of the Ontario Provincial Board of Health.

9. The "picture" referred to is contained in Crozier's book, My Inner Life: Being a Chapter in Personal Evolution and Autobiography *(1898). Crozier graduated from the University of Toronto in 1872; among his classmates were Dick Zimmerman and William Osler (the latter for two years only, at which time he left to attend McGill).*

the least part of an education, and, as I recall them, our teachers in their life and doctrine set forth a true and lively word to the great enlightenment of our darkness. They stand out in the background of my memory as a group of men whose influence and example were most helpful. In William R. Beaumont [10] and Edward Mulberry Hodder,[11] we had before us the highest type of the cultivated English surgeon. In Henry H. Wright [12] we saw the incarnation of faithful devotion to duty—too faithful, we thought, as we trudged up to the eight o'clock lecture in the morning. In W. T. Aikins [13] a practical surgeon of remarkable skill and an ideal teacher for the general practitioner. How we wondered and delighted in the anatomical demonstrations of Dr. Richardson, whose infective enthusiasm did much to make anatomy the favorite subject among the students. I had the double advantage of attending the last course of Dr. Ogden and the first of Dr. Thorburn on materia medica and therapeutics. And Dr. Oldright had just begun his career of unselfish devotion to the cause of hygiene.

To one of my teachers I must pay in passing the tribute of filial affection. There are men here today who feel as I do about Dr. James Bovell [14]—that he was one of those finer spirits, not uncommon in life, touched to finer issues only in a suitable environment.

10. *William R. Beaumont (1803–1875), born and educated in London, came to Canada in 1841 and taught surgery and ophthalmic surgery in Toronto. In 1836 he invented an instrument for suturing which some writers claim was the basis for one part of Singer's sewing machine.*

11. *Edward M. Hodder (1810–1878) was born in Kent, England. He received his degree in London in 1834 and over the next four years practiced there and in France. In 1838 he came to Canada and in 1843 to Toronto, where he practiced as a surgeon and gynecologist until his death. From 1870 on he was Dean of the Toronto School of Medicine.*

12. *Henry Hover Wright (1816–1899) was much associated with Dr. John Rolph, who was an instigator of the Rebellion of 1837; Wright, then a medical student, played a key role in helping Rolph escape to the United States when the rebellion collapsed. Wright was Professor of Medicine in the University of Toronto for many years, and was noted for his excellent teaching and for his honesty.*

13. *William T. Aikins (1827–1895) was born near Toronto and educated in Ontario and at Philadelphia, where he received his M.D. in 1850. Immediately thereafter he became involved with medical education and medical politics in Toronto. He practiced as a surgeon and was an early Canadian exponent of Listerism.*

14. *James Bovell (1817–1880) was one of the three teachers whom Osler most revered, and to whom he dedicated his famous textbook, The Prin-*

Would the Paul of evolution have been Thomas Henry Huxley had the Senate elected the young naturalist to a chair in this university in 1851? Only men of a certain metal rise superior to their surroundings, and while Dr. Bovell had that all-important combination of boundless ambition with energy and industry, he had that fatal fault of diffuseness, in which even genius gets strangled. With a quadrilateral mind, which he kept spinning like a teetotum, one side was never kept uppermost for long at a time. Caught in the storm which shook the scientific world with the publication of the "Origin of Species," instead of sailing before the wind, even were it with bare poles, he put about and sought a harbor of refuge in writing a work on Natural Theology, which you will find on the shelves of second-hand bookshops in a company made respectable at least by the presence of Paley.[15] He was an omnivorous reader and transmuter, he could talk pleasantly, even at times transcendentally, upon anything in the science of the day, from protoplasm to evolution; but he lacked concentration and that scientific accuracy which only comes with a long training (sometimes indeed never comes), and which is the ballast of the boat. But the bent of his mind was devotional, and early swept into the Tractarian movement, he became an advanced Churchman, a good Anglican Catholic. As he

ciples and Practice of Medicine. *This long paragraph pays eloquent tribute to Bovell's memory.*

15. William Paley (1743–1805), Archdeacon of Carlisle. The reference is to Paley's Natural Theology; or Evidence of the Existence and Attributes of the Deity Collected from the Appearances of Nature, 1802. *This book provides a classic example of teleological reasoning; it was well received and widely read until Darwin's work revealed its essential weakness.*

chaffingly remarked one day to his friend, the Reverend Mr. Darling, he was like the waterman in "Pilgrim's Progress," rowing one way, towards Rome, but looking steadfastly in the other direction, towards Lambeth. His "Steps to the Altar," and his "Lectures on the Advent" attest the earnestness of his convictions; and later in life, following the example of Linacre, he took orders and became another illustration of what Cotton Mather calls the angelical conjunction of medicine with divinity. Then, how well I recall the keen love with which he would engage in metaphysical discussions, and the ardor with which he studied Kant, Hamilton, Reed and Mill. At that day to the Rev. Prof. Bevan was entrusted the rare privilege of directing the minds of the thinking youths at the Provincial University into proper philosophical channels. It was rumored that the hungry sheep looked up and were not fed. I thought so at least, for certain of them, led by T. Wesley Mills,[16] came over daily after Dr. Bovell's four o'clock lecture to reason high and long with him

"On Providence, Foreknowledge, Will, and Fate—
Fixed Fate, Freewill, Foreknowledge absolute." [17]

Yet withal his main business in life was as a physician, much sought after for his skill in diag-

16. T. Wesley Mills (1847–1915) and Osler were students together in Toronto, 1867 to 1869, and later they taught together at McGill. Mills was a physiologist and a veterinarian, and also energetically applied himself to the study of music. He published books and papers in all three fields.

17. ". . . In discourse more sweet

.   .   .   .   .

Others apart sat on a Hill retir'd,
In thoughts more elevate, and reason'd high
Of Providence, Foreknowledge, Will, and Fate,
Fixt Fate, free-will, foreknowledge absolute,
And found no end, in wand'ring mazes lost."
(Milton, Paradise Lost, Bk. II, lines 555–561.)

nosis, and much beloved for his loving heart. He had been brought up in the very best practical schools. A pupil of Bright and of Addison, a warm personal friend of Stokes and of Graves, he maintained loyally the traditions of Guy's and taught us to reverence his great masters. As a teacher, he had grasped the fundamental truth announced by John Hunter of the unity of physiological and pathological processes, and, as became the occupant of the chair of the Institute of Medicine, he would discourse on pathological processes in lectures on physiology, and illustrate the physiology of bioplasm in lectures on the pathology of tumors to the bewilderment of the students. When in September, 1870, he wrote to me that he did not intend to return from the West Indies, I felt that I had lost a father and a friend; but in Robert Palmer Howard,[18] of Montreal, I found a noble step-father, and to these two men, and to my first teacher, the Rev. W. A. Johnson,[19] of Weston, I owe my success in life —if success means getting what you want and being satisfied with it.

18. Robert Palmer Howard (1823–1889) was Osler's teacher and mentor at McGill, and for him Osler displayed a truly filial affection. Howard was a distinguished physician and served as Professor of Medicine and Dean of the Faculty of Medicine, McGill.

19. Rev. W. A. Johnson (1816–1880) first stirred in Osler a genuine interest in natural science, thus unwittingly playing some role in turning Osler from the ministry to medicine. Johnson was headmaster at Trinity College School, a sort of private high school, in Weston, Ontario; Osler attended for eighteen months before attending the university, where he began studying for the ministry but soon changed his resolve to medicine.

II

*O*f the value of an introductory lecture I am not altogether certain. I do not remember to have derived any enduring benefit from the many that I have been called upon to hear, or from the not a few I have inflicted in my day. On the whole I am in favor of abolishing the old custom, but as this is a very special occasion, with special addresses, I consider myself most happy to have been selected for this part of the programme. To the audience at large I fear that much of what I have to say will appear trite and commonplace, but bear with me, since, indeed, to most of you how good soever the word, the season is long past in which it could be spoken to your edification. As I glance from face to face the most striking single peculiarity is the extraordinary diversity that exists among you. Alike in that you are men and white, you are unlike in your features, very unlike in your minds and in your mental training, and your teachers will mourn the singular inequalities in your capacities. And so it is sad to think what will be your careers. For one success, for another failure; one will tread the primrose path to the great bonfire,[20] another the

20. *"I had thought to have let in some of all professions that go the primrose way to the everlasting bon-fire"* (*Porter, in* Macbeth, *Act 2, Scene 3*).

straight and narrow way to renown; some of the best of you will be stricken early on the road, and will join that noble band of youthful martyrs who loved not their lives to the death; others, perhaps the most brilliant among you, like my old friend and comrade, Dick Zimmerman [21] (how he would have rejoiced to see this day!), the Fates will overtake and whirl to destruction just as success seems assured. When the iniquity of oblivion has blindly scattered her poppy over us, some of you will be the trusted counsellors of this community, and the heads of departments in this Faculty while for the large majority of you, let us hope, is reserved the happiest and most useful lot given to man —to become vigorous, whole-souled, intelligent general practitioners.

It seems a bounden duty on such an occasion to be honest and frank, so I propose to tell you the secret of life as I have seen the game played, and as I have tried to play it myself. You remember in one of the "Jungle Stories," that when Mowgli wished to be avenged on the villagers he could only get the help of Hathi and his sons by sending them the master-word. [22] This I propose to give you in the hope, yes, the full assurance, that some of you at least will lay hold upon it to your profit. Though a little one, the master-word looms large in meaning. It is the open sesame to every portal,

21. Richard Zimmerman (1851–1888) led his class at the Toronto School of Medicine; he began practice in Toronto in 1874. He became a demonstrator in histology, a pathologist, and a surgeon; his apparently brilliant prospects ended abruptly with his sudden death at age 37.

22. "'But, indeed, and truly, Little Brother, it is not—it is not seemly to say "Come," and "Go," to Hathi. Remember, he is the Master of the Jungle, and before the Man-Pack changed the look on thy face, he taught thee a Master-word of the Jungle.'
"'That is all over. I have a Master-word for him now. Bid him come to Mowgli, the Frog, and if he does not hear at first, bid him come because of the Sack of the Fields of Bhurtpore.'" (Rudyard Kipling, The Jungle Book, "Letting in the Jungle").

the great equalizer in the world,
the true philosopher's stone which
transmutes all the base metal of
humanity into gold. The stupid
man among you it will make
bright, the bright man brilliant,
and the brilliant student steady.
With the magic word in your
heart all things are possible, and
without it all study is vanity and
vexation. The miracles of life are
with it; the blind see by touch, the
deaf hear with eyes, the dumb
speak with fingers. To the youth
it brings hope, to the middle-aged
confidence, to the aged repose.
True balm of hurt minds, in its
presence the heart of the sorrow-
ful is lightened and consoled. It is
directly responsible for all advances in medicine during the past
twenty-five centuries. Laying hold
upon it. Hippocrates made obser-
vation and science the warp and
woof of our art. Galen so read its
meaning that fifteen centuries
stopped thinking, and slept until
awakened by the *De Fabrica* of
Vesalius, which is the very incarnation of the master-word. With
its inspiration Harvey gave an impulse to a larger circulation than
he wot of, an impulse which we
feel to-day. Hunter sounded all its
heights and depths, and stands out
in our history as one of the great
exemplars of its virtues. With it
Virchow smote the rock and the
waters of progress gushed out;
while in the hands of Pasteur it
proved a very talisman to open to
us a new heaven in medicine and

a new earth in surgery. Not only has it been the touchstone of progress, but it is the measure of success in everyday life. Not a man before you but is beholden to it for his position here, while he who addresses you has that honor directly in consequence of having had it graven on his heart when he was as you are to-day. And the Master-Word is *Work*, a little one, as I have said, but fraught with momentous sequences if you can but write it on the tables of your heart, and bind it upon your forehead. But there is a serious difficulty in getting you to understand the paramount importance of the work-habit as part of your organization. You are not far from the Tom Sawyer stage with its philosophy "that work consists of whatever a body is obliged to do, and play consists of whatever a body is not obliged to do."[23]

A great many hard things may be said of the work-habit. For many of us it means a hard battle; the few take to it naturally; the many prefer idleness and never learn to love to labor. Listen to this: "Look at one of your industrious fellows for a moment, I beseech you," says Robert Louis Stevenson.[24] "He sows hurry and reaps indigestion; he puts a vast deal of activity out to interest, and receives a large measure of nervous derangement in return. Either he absents himself entirely from all fellowship, and lives a recluse in a garret, with carpet slippers

23. *"[Tom] had discovered a great law of human action, without knowing it—namely, that in order to make a man or a boy covet a thing, it is only necessary to make the thing difficult to attain. If he had been a great and wise philosopher, like the writer of this book, he would now have comprehended that Work consists of whatever a body is* obliged *to do and that Play consists of whatever a body is* not obliged *to do"* (Mark Twain, Tom Sawyer, *Ch. 2, 1876*).

24. *"Consequently, if a person cannot be happy without remaining idle, idle he should remain. It is a revolutionary precept; but thanks to hunger and the workhouse, one not easily to be abused. . . . Look at one of your industrious fellows [etc.: Osler cites the remainder of the passage verbatim]"* (Virginibus Puerisque, *"An Apology for Idlers," 1882*).
"Soon, soon, it seems to you, you must come forth on some conspicuous hilltop, and but a little way farther, against the setting sun, descry the spires of El Dorado. Little do ye know your own blessedness; for to travel hopefully is a better thing than to arrive, and the true success is to labour" (Virginibus Puerisque, *"El Dorado," 1882*).

and a leaden inkpot; or he comes among people swiftly and bitterly, in a contraction of his whole nervous system, to discharge some temper before he returns to work. I do not care how much or how well he works, this fellow is an evil feature in other people's lives." These are the sentiments of an overworked, dejected man; let me quote the motto of his saner moments: "To travel hopeful is better than to arrive, and the true success is in labor." If you wish to learn of the miseries of scholars in order to avoid them, read Part I, Section 2, Member 3, Subsection XV, of that immortal work, the "Anatomy of Melancholy,"[25] but I am here to warn you against these evils, and to entreat you to form good habits in your student days.

At the outset, appreciate clearly the aims and objects each one of you should have in view—a knowledge of disease and its cure, and a knowledge of yourselves. The one, a special education, will make you a practitioner of medicine; the other, an inner education, may make you a truly good man, four-square and without flaw. The one is extrinsic and is largely accomplished by teacher and tutor, by text and by tongue; the other is intrinsic and is the mental salvation to be wrought by each one for himself. The first may be had without the second; any one of you may become an active practitioner, without ever having had

25. "*. . . hard students are commonly troubled with gouts, catarrhs, rheums, cachexia, bradypepsia, bad eyes, stone, and colic, crudities, oppilations, vertigo, winds, consumptions, and all such diseases as come by overmuch sitting; they are most part lean, dry, ill-coloured, spend their fortunes, lose their wits, and many times their lives, and all through immoderate pains and extraordinary studies. . . .*"

sense enough to realize that through life you have been a fool; or you may have the second without the first, and, without knowing much of the art, you may have the endowments of head and heart that make the little you do possess go very far in the community. With what I hope to infect you is the desire to have a due proportion of each.

So far as your professional education is concerned, what I shall say may make for each one of you an easy path easier. The multiplicity of the subjects to be studied is a difficulty, and it is hard for teacher and student to get a due sense of proportion in the work. We are in a transition stage in our methods of teaching, and we have not everywhere got away from the idea of the examination as the "be-all and end-all;" so that the student has continually before his eyes the magical letters of the degree he seeks. And this is well, perhaps, if you will remember that having, in the old phrase, commenced Bachelor of Medicine, you have only reached a point from which you can begin a life-long process of education.

So many and varied are the aspects presented by this theme that I can only lay stress upon a few of the more essential. The very first step towards success in any occupation is to become interested in it. Locke put this in a very happy way when he said, give a pupil "a relish of knowledge,"[26] and you put life into his work. And there is nothing more certain than that you cannot study well if you are not interested in your profession. Your presence here is a warrant that in some way you have become attracted to the study of medicine, but the speculative possibilities so warmly cherished at the outset are apt to cool when in contact with the stern realities of the class-room. Most of you have already experienced the all-absorbing attraction of the scientific branches, and nowadays the practical method of presentation has given a zest which was usually lacking in the old theoretical teaching. The life has become more serious in consequence, and medical students have put away many of the childish tricks with which we used to keep up their bad name. Compare the picture of the "sawbones" of 1842, as given in the recent biography of Sir Henry Acland,[27] with their representatives to-day, and it is evident a great revolution has been effected, and very largely by the salutary influence of improved methods of education. It is possible now to fill out a day with practical work, varied enough to prevent monotony, and so arranged that the knowledge is picked out by the student himself, not thrust into him, willy-nilly, at the point of the tongue. He exercises his wits, and is no longer a passive Strassbourg goose, tied up and stuffed to repletion.

26. *I have not found precisely these words in Locke, but in* An Essay Concerning Human Understanding, *Book II, Chapter XXI, Section 71 ("We can change the agreeableness or disagreeableness in things"), he uses the metaphor repeatedly. "The relish of the mind is as various as that of the body, and like that too may be altered. . . ." And again: "Fashion and the common opinion have settled wrong notions, and education and custom ill habits, the just values of things are misplaced, and the palates of men corrupted. Pains should be taken to rectify these; and contrary habits change our pleasures, and give a relish to that which is necessary or conducive to our happiness."*

27. *The book is by J. B. Atlay:* Sir Henry Wentworth Acland, Bart. K.C.B., F.R.S., Regius Professor of Medicine in the University of Oxford. A Memoir . . . with Portraits and Illustrations (1903). *Acland (1815–1900) was succeeded as Regius Professor by Sir Burdon Sanderson, who was in turn succeeded by Osler. It was in Acland's library that Osler first saw the paintings, on a panel, of Linacre, Harvey, and Sydenham. Noting his excitement over these portraits, Mrs. Osler later arranged to have them copied, and she gave them to Osler on his birthday.*

How can you take the greatest possible advantage of your capacities with the least possible strain? By cultivating system. I say cultivating advisedly, since some of you will find the acquisition of systematic habits very hard. There are minds congenitally systematic; others have a life-long fight against an inherited tendency to diffuseness and carelessness in work. A few brilliant fellows try to dispense with it altogether, but they are a burden to their brethren and a sore trial to their intimates. I have heard it remarked that order is the badge of an ordinary mind. So it may be, but as practitioners of medicine we have to be thankful to get into this useful class. Let me entreat those of you who are here for the first time to lay to heart what I say on this matter. Forget all else, but take away this counsel of a man who has had to fight a hard battle, but not always a successful one, for the little order he has had in his life: take away with you a profound conviction of the value of system in your work. I appeal to the freshmen especially, because you to-day make a beginning, and your future career depends very much upon the habits you will form during this session. To follow the routine of the classes is easy enough, but to take routine into every part of your daily life is a hard task. Some of you will start out joyfully as did Christian and Hopeful,[28] and for many days will journey safely towards the De-

28. The Pilgrim's Progress (1678), by John Bunyan (1628–1688) is an allegory, recapitulating symbolically Bunyan's conversion as a Puritan.

lectable Mountains, dreaming of them and not thinking of disaster until you find yourselves in the strong captivity of Doubt and under the grinding tyranny of Despair. You have been over-confident. Begin again and more cautiously. No student escapes wholly from these perils and trials; be not disheartened, expect them. Let each hour of the day have its allotted duty, and culti-vate that power of concentration which grows with its exercise, so that the attention neither flags nor wavers, but settles with a bull-dog tenacity on the subject before you. Constant repetition makes a good habit fit easily in your mind, and by the end of the session you may have gained that most precious of all knowledge—the power to work. Do not underestimate the difficulty you will have in wringing from your reluctant selves the stern de-termination to exact the uttermost minute on your schedule. Do not get too interested in one study at the expense of another, but so map out your day that due allowance is given to each. Only in this way can the average student get the best that he can out of his capaci-ties. And it is worth all the pains and trouble he can possibly take for the ultimate gain—if he can reach his doctorate with system so ingrained that it has become an integral part of his being. The artistic sense of perfection in work is another much-to-be-desired qual-ity to be cultivated. No matter how trifling the matter on hand, do it with a feeling that it demands the best that is in you, and when done look it over with a critical eye, not sparing a strict judgment on yourself. This it is that makes anatomy a student's touchstone. Take the man who does his "part" to perfection, who has got out all there is in it, who labors over the tags of connective tissue, and who demonstrates Meckel's ganglion [29] in his part—this is the fellow in after years who is apt in emergencies, who saves a leg badly smashed in a railway accident, or fights out to the finish, never knowing when he is beaten, in a case of typhoid fever.

Learn to love the freedom of the student life, only too quickly to pass away; the absence of the coarser cares of after days, the joy of comradeship, the delight in new work, the happiness in knowing that you are making progress. Once only can you enjoy these pleasures. The seclusion of the student life is not always good for a man, particularly for those of you who will afterwards engage in general practice, since you will miss that facility of intercourse upon which often the doctor's success depends. On the other hand, sequestration is essential for those of you with high ambitions proportionate to your capacity. It was for such that St. Chrysostom [30] gave his famous counsel, "Depart from the highways and transplant thyself into some enclosed ground, for it

29. *The sphenopalatine ganglion.*

30. *Saint John Chrysostom (c.347–407) was a brilliant orator, named patriarch of Constantinople in 398. Reportedly, he often had to chide the congregation for applauding in church.*

is hard for a tree that stands by the wayside to keep its fruit till it be ripe."

Has work no dangers connected with it? What of this bogey of overwork of which we hear so much? There are dangers, but they may readily be avoided with a little care. I can only mention two, one physical, one mental. The very best students are often not the strongest. Ill-health, the bridle of Theages, as Plato called it in the case of one of his friends whose mind had thriven at the expense of the body,[31] may have been the diverting influence toward books or the profession. Among the good men who have studied with me there stand out in my remembrance many a young Lycidas,[32] "dead ere his prime," sacrificed to carelessness in habits of living and neglect of ordinary sanitary laws. Medical students are much exposed to infection of all sorts, to combat which the body must be kept in first-class condition. Grossteste, the great Bishop of Lincoln,[33] remarked that there were three things necessary for temporal salvation—food, sleep, and a cheerful disposition. Add to these suitable exercise and you have the means by which good health may be maintained. Not that health is to be a matter of perpetual solicitude, but habits which favor the *corpus sanum* foster the *mens sana*, in which the joy of living and the joy of working are blended in one harmony. Let me read you a quo-

31. *Despite diligent search I cannot identify this reference.*

32. *Lycidas is the name of the shepherd in Virgil's* Eclogue, *and Milton used this name in his famous elegy celebrating the untimely death of Edward King, a Cambridge Fellow who drowned in 1637.*
"For Lycidas *is dead, dead ere his prime,*
Young Lycidas, *and hath not left his peer."*
33. *Robert Grosteste (1175?–1253), Bishop of London, 1235–1253. He witnessed the confirmation of the Magna Charta in 1236. He has been described as ". . . a manifest confuter of the pope and the king, the blamer of prelates, the corrector of monks, the director of priests, the instructor of clerks, the support of scholars, the preacher to the people, the persecutor of the incontinent, the sedulous student of all scripture, the hammer and the despiser of the Romans"* (Dictionary of National Biography).

tation from old Burton, the great authority on *morbi eruditorum*. There are "many reasons why students dote more often than others. The first is their negligence. Other men look to their tools: a painter will wash his pencils; a smith will look to his hammer, anvil, forge; a husbandman will mend his plough-irons, and grind his hatchet, if it be dull; a falconer or huntsman will have an especial care of his hawks, hounds, horses, dogs, etc.; a musician will string and unstring his lute, etc.; only scholars neglect that instrument, their brain and spirits (I mean) which they daily use." [34]

Much study is not only believed to be a weariness of the flesh, but also an active cause of ill-health of mind, in all grades and phase. I deny that work, legitimate work, has anything to do with this. It is that foul fiend Worry who is responsible for a large majority of the cases. The more carefully one looks into the cause of nervous breakdown in students, the less important is work *per se* as a factor. There are a few cases of genuine overwork, but they are not common. Of the causes of worry in the student life there are three of prime importance to which I may briefly refer.

An anticipatory attitude of mind, a perpetual forecasting, disturbs the even tenor of his way and leads to disaster. Years ago a sentence in one of Carlyle's essays made a lasting impression on me:

34. *Robert Burton (1577–1640).* Anatomy of Melancholy, *Pt. I, Sec. 2, Mem. 3, Subs. 15.*

"Our duty is not to *see* what lies dimly at a distance, but to *do* what lies clearly at hand." [35] I have long maintained that the best motto for a student is, "Take no thought for the morrow." Let the day's work suffice; live for it, regardless of what the future has in store, believing that to-morrow should take thought for the things of itself. There is no such safeguard against the morbid apprehensions about the future, the dread of examinations and the doubt of ultimate success. Nor is there any risk that such an attitude may breed carelessness. On the contrary, the absorption in the duty of the hour is in itself the best guarantee of ultimate success. "He that regardeth the wind shall not sow, and he that observeth the clouds shall not reap,"[36] which means you cannot work profitably with your mind set upon the future.

Another potent cause of worry is an idolatry by which many of you will be sore let and hindered. The mistress of your studies should be the heavenly Aphrodite, the motherless daughter of Uranus. Give her your whole heart and she will be your protectress and friend. A jealous creature, brooking no second, if she finds you trifling and coquetting with her rival, the younger, early Aphrodite, daughter of Zeus and Dione, she will whistle you off, and let you down the wind to be a prey, perhaps to the examiners, certainly to the worm regret. In plainer language,

35. *"Happy men are full of the present, for its bounty suffices them; and wise men also, for its duties engage them. Our grand business undoubtedly is, not to see what lies dimly at a distance, but to do what lies clearly at hand"* (Signs of the Times, 1829). *Carlyle returned to this theme later: "Do the duty that lies nearest thee"* (Sartor Resartus, 1833).

36. *"He that observeth the wind shall not sow; and he that regardeth the clouds shall not reap"* (Ecclesiastes 11:4).

put your affections in cold storage for a few years, and you will take them out ripened, perhaps a bit mellow, but certainly less subject to those frequent changes which perplex so many young men. Only a grand passion, an all-absorbing devotion to the elder goddess, can save the man with a congenital tendency to philandering, the flighty Lydgate who sports with Celia and Dorothea, and upon whom the judgment ultimately falls in a basilplant of a wife like Rosamond.[37]

And thirdly, one and all of you will have to face the ordeal of every student in this generation who sooner or later tries to mix the waters of science with the oil of faith. You can have a great deal of both if you can only keep them separate. The worry comes from the attempt at mixture. As general practitioners you will need all the faith you can carry, and while it may not always be of the conventional pattern, when expressed in your lives rather than on your lips, the variety is not a bad one from the standpoint of St. James, and may help to counteract the common scandal alluded to in the celebrated diary of that gossipy old parson-doctor, the Rev. John Ward:[38] "One told the Bishop of Gloucester that he imagined physitians of all men the most competent judges of all others' affairs of religion—and his reason was because they were wholly unconcerned with it."

37. *Dr. Lydgate was the physician (purportedly based on Sir Henry Acland) in George Eliot's* Middlemarch *(1871). Dorothea Brooke, the heroine, was a wealthy widow who supports Lydgate's medical reforms; Celia Brooke, Dorothea's sister; Rosamond Vincy, selfish and ambitious, was the young lady who became Mrs. Lydgate.*

38. *John Ward (1629–1681) studied at Oxford, receiving an M.A. in 1652. In 1662 he became vicar of Stratford-upon-Avon. Between 1648 and 1679 he maintained intermittently a commonplace book. Some portions were published in the nineteenth and some in the twentieth centuries.*

III

*P*rofessional work of any sort tends to narrow the mind, to limit the point of view, and to put a hall-mark on a man of a most unmistakable kind. On the one hand are the intense, ardent natures, absorbed in their studies and quickly losing interest in everything but their profession, while other faculties and interests "fust" unused. On the other hand are the bovine brethren, who think of nothing but the treadmill and the corn. From very different causes, the one from concentration, the other from apathy, both are apt to neglect those outside studies that widen the sympathies and help a man to get the best there is out of life. Like art, medicine is an exacting mistress, and in the pursuit of one of the scientific branches, sometimes, too, in practice, not a portion of a man's spirit may be left free for other distractions, but this does not often happen. On account of the intimate personal nature of his work, the medical man, perhaps more than any other man, needs that higher education of which Plato speaks, "that education in virtue from youth upwards, which enables a man eagerly to pursue the ideal perfection."[39] It is not for all, nor can all attain to it, but

39. *"For we are not speaking of education in this narrower sense, but of that other education in virtue from youth upwards, which makes a man eagerly pursue the ideal perfection of citizenship, and teaches him how rightly to rule and how to obey. This is the only education which, upon our view, deserves the name"* (Plato, Laws I).

there is comfort and help in the pursuit, even though the end is never reached. For a large majority the daily round and the common task furnished more than enough to satisfy their heart's desire, and there seems no room left for anything else. Like the good, easy man whom Milton [40] scores in the Areopagitica, whose religion was a "traffic so entangled that of all mysteries he could not skill to keep a stock going upon that trade," and handed it over with all the locks and keys to "a divine of note and estimation," so is it with many of us in the matter of this higher education. No longer intrinsic, wrought in us and ingrained, it has become, in Milton's phrase, a "dividual movable," handed over nowadays to the daily press or to the hap-hazard instruction of the pulpit, the platform, or the magazines. Like a good many other things, it comes to a better and more enduring form if not too consciously sought. The all-important thing is to get a relish for the good company of the race in a daily intercourse with some of the great minds of all ages. Now, in the spring-time of life, pick your intimates among them, and begin a systematic cultivation of their works. Many of you will need a strong leaven to raise you above the level of the dough in which it will be your lot to labor. Uncongenial surroundings, an ever-present dissonance between the aspirations within and the ac-

40. *"A wealthy man, addicted to his pleasure and to his profits, finds religion to be a traffic so entangled, and of so many piddling accounts, that of all mysteries he cannot skill to keep a stock going upon that trade. What should he do? fain he would have the name to be religious, fain he would bear up with his neighbours in that. What does he therefore, but resolve to give over toiling, and to find himself out some factor, to whose care and credit he may commit the whole managing of his religious affairs? some Divine of note and estimation that must be. To him he adheres, resigns the whole warehouse of his religion, with all the locks and keys, into his custody; and indeed makes the very person of that man his religion; esteems his associating with him a sufficient evidence and commendatory of his own piety. So that a man may say his religion is now no more within himself, but is become a dividual movable, and goes and comes near him, according as that good man frequents the house"* (*John Milton, Areopagitica, 1644*).

tualities without, the oppressive discords of human society, the bitter tragedies of life, the *lacrymae rerum*,[41] beside the hidden springs of which we sit in sad despair—all these tend to foster in some natures a cynicism quite foreign to our vocation, and to which this inner education offers the best antidote. Personal contact with men of high purpose and character will help a man to make a start—to have the desire, at least, but in its fulness this culture—for that word best expresses it—has to be wrought by each one for himself. Start at once a bed-side library [42] and spend the last half hour of the day in communion with the saints of humanity. There are great lessons to be learned from Job and from David, from Isaiah and St. Paul. Taught by Shakespeare you may take your intellectual and moral measure with singular precision. Learn to love Epictetus and Marcus Aurelius. Should you be so fortunate as to be born a Platonist, Jowett will introduce you to the great master through whom alone we can think in certain levels, and whose perpetual modernness startles and delights. Montaigne will teach moderation in all things, and to be "sealed of his tribe" is a special privilege. We have in the profession only a few great literary heroes of the first rank, the friendship and counsel of two of whom you cannot too earnestly seek. Sir Thomas Browne's "Religio Medici" [43] should be your

41. The reference is to Virgil's Aeneid (Bk. I, lines 460–462): Sunt lacrymae rerum, et mentem mortalia tangunt. "There are tears for what befalls, and hearts touched by the chances of mortality." The phrase alludes to the innate sadness of human life.

42. Osler's personal selection of his essays, Aequanimitas, *has carried the following list in every edition except the first; Sir William suggested that these are "books which you may make close friends."*

    I. Old and New Testament.
    II. Shakespeare.
    III. Montaigne.
    IV. Plutarch's Lives.
    V. Marcus Aurelius.
    VI. Epictetus.
    VII. Religio Medici.
    VIII. Don Quixote.
    IX. Emerson.
    X. Oliver Wendell Holmes: Breakfast-Table Series

43. Sir Thomas Browne (1605–1682) without question was Osler's favorite author, and the Religio Medici *provided inspiration and solace throughout his life until the last moment and perhaps beyond: on the velvet pall over his bier lay a single sheaf of lilies and his favorite copy of the* Religio. *The book "is a 'memorial' intended to record for the author's further use, rather than his present satisfaction, a sum of personal views resulting from temper and experience, written at the sober age of thirty . . ." (Jean Jacques Denonain, Introduction to* Religio Medici, *Cambridge, The University Press, 1966).*

pocket companion, while from the "Breakfast-Table Series" of Oliver Wendell Holmes [44] you can glean a philosophy of life peculiarly suited to the needs of a physician. There are at least a dozen or more works which would be helpful in getting that wisdom in life which only comes to those who earnestly seek it.

A conscientious pursuit of Plato's ideal perfection may teach you the three great lessons of life. You may learn to consume your own smoke.[45] The atmosphere of life is darkened by the murmurings and whimperings of men and women over the non-essentials, the trifles, that are inevitably incident to the hurly-burly of the day's routine. Things cannot always go your way. Learn to accept in silence the minor aggravations, cultivate the gift of taciturnity and consume your own smoke with an extra draught of hard work, so that those about you may not be annoyed with the dust and soot of your complaints. More than any other the practitioner of medicine may illustrate the second great lesson, that we are here not to get all we can out of life for ourselves, but to try to make the lives of others happier. This is the essence of the oft-repeated admonition of Christ, "He that findeth his life shall lose it, and he that loseth his life for my sake shall find it," [46] on which hard saying if the children of this generation would lay hold, there would be less misery and discontent in the

44. The Autocrat of the Breakfast-Table (*1858*), The Professor at the Breakfast-Table (*1859*), *and* The Poet at the Breakfast-Table (*1869*). *Holmes' essays, both witty and serious, first appeared in the* Atlantic Monthly; *he was a practicing physician, a professor of anatomy, Dean of Harvard Medical School, and a noted lecturer and essayist both on science and on literature. He was the author of "The Wonderful One-Hoss Shay."*

45. *"The first lesson of literature, no less than of life, is the learning how to burn your own smoke" (J. R. Lowell [1819–1891], My Study Windows, 1870 p. 228).*

46. *Matthew 10:39, 16:25; Mark 8:35; Luke 9:24.*

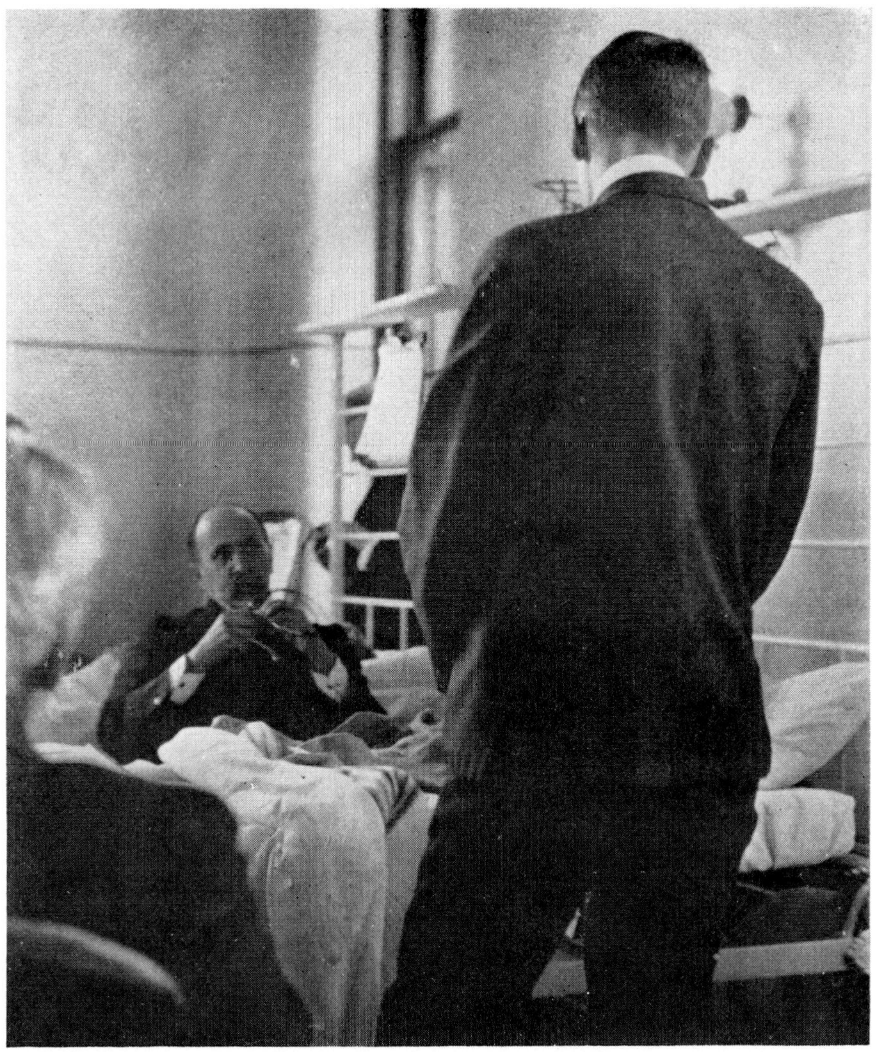

Osler at the bedside, Johns Hopkins Hospital. (Courtesy National Library of Medicine, Bethesda, Maryland.)

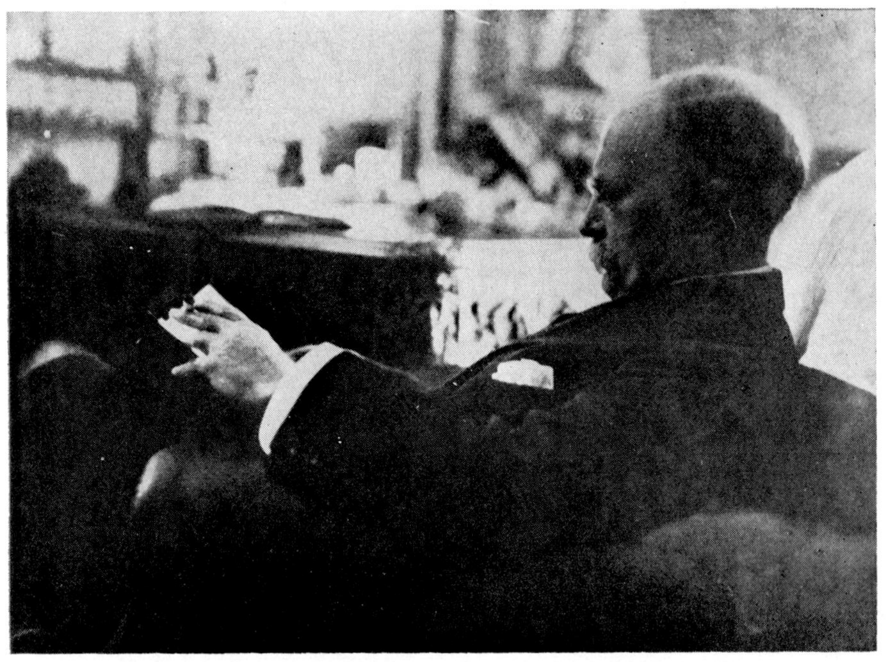

Osler reading in his study at Oxford. (Courtesy Osler Library, McGill University, Montreal.)

world. It is not possible for anyone to have better opportunities to live this lesson than you will enjoy. The practice of medicine is an art, not a trade, a calling, not a business, a calling in which your heart will be exercised equally with your head. Often the best part of your work will have nothing to do with potions and powders, but with the exercise of an influence of the strong upon the weak, of the righteous upon the wicked, the wise upon the foolish. To you as the trusted family counsellor the father will come with his anxieties, the mother with her hidden griefs, the daughter with her trials, and the son with his follies. Fully one-third of the work you do will be entered in other books than yours. Courage and cheerfulness will not only carry you over the rough places of life, but will enable you to bring comfort and help to the weak-hearted, and will console you in the sad hours when, like Uncle Toby, you have "to whistle that you may not weep." [47]

And the third great lesson you may learn is the hardest of all— that the law of the higher life is only fulfilled by love or charity. Many a physician whose daily work is a daily round of benefi- cence will say hard things and will think hard thoughts of a colleague. No sin will so easily beset you as uncharitableness towards your brother practitioner. So strong is the personal element in the prac- tice of medicine, and so many are

47. *Mr. Toby Shandy, uncle of Tris- tram Shandy: "My uncle Toby would never offer to answer this by any other kind of argument, than that of whistling half a dozen bars of Lilla- bullero.—You must know it was the usual channel thro' which his passions got vent . . ." (Laurence Sterne [1713–1768], Tristram Shandy, Bk. 1, Ch. 21).*

the wagging tongues in every par-
ish, that evil speaking, lying and
slandering find a shining mark in
the lapses and mistakes which are
inevitable in our work. There is no
reason for discord and disagree-
ment, and the only way to avoid
trouble is to have two plain rules.
From the day you begin practice
never under any circumstances
listen to a tale told to the detri-
ment of a brother practitioner.
And when any dispute or trouble
does arise, go frankly, ere sunset,
and talk the matter over, in which
way you may gain a brother and
a friend. Very easy to carry out,
you may think! Far from it;
there is no harder battle to fight.
Theoretically, there seems to be
no difficulty, but when the concrete
wound is rankling, and after Mrs.
Jones has rubbed in the cayenne
pepper by declaring that Dr. J.
told her in confidence of your
shocking bungling, your attitude
of mind is that you would rather
see him in purgatory than make
advances towards reconciliation.
Wait until the day of your trial
comes and then remember my
words.

And in closing may I say a few
words to the younger practitioners
in the audience whose activities will
wax, not wane, with the growing
years of the century which opens
so auspiciously for this school, for
this city, for this country. You en-
ter a noble heritage, made by no
efforts of your own, but by genera-
tions of men who have unselfishly

sought to do the best they could for suffering mankind. Much has been done, much remains to do; a way has been opened, and to the possibilities in the scientific development of medicine there seems to be no limit. Except in its application, as general practitioners, you will not have much to do with this. Yours is a higher and a more sacred duty. Think not to light a light to shine before men that they may see your good works; contrariwise, you belong to the great army of quiet workers, physicians and priests, sisters and nurses, all over the world, the members of which strive not neither do they cry, nor are their voices heard in the streets, but to them is given the ministry of consolation in sorrow, need and sickness. Like the ideal wife of whom Plutarch speaks,[48] the best doctor is often the one of whom the public hears least; but nowadays in the fierce light that beats upon the hearth, it is increasingly difficult to live the secluded life in which our best work is done. To you the silent workers of the ranks, in villages and country districts, in the slums of our great cities, in the mining camps and factory towns, in the homes of the rich and in the hovels of the poor—to you is given the harder task of illustrating in your lives the old Hippocratic standards of learning, of sagacity, of humanity and of probity. Of learning, that you may apply in your practice the best that is known in our art, and that with

48. *Like the earlier reference to Plato, I have been unable to trace this allusion.*

the increase of that priceless endowment of sagacity, so that to
all everywhere skilled succor may
come in the hour of urgent need.
Of a humanity that will show in
your daily life tenderness and con-
sideration to the weak, infinite pity
to the suffering and a broad charity
to all. Of a probity that will make
you under all circumstances true
to yourselves, true to your high
calling, and true to your fellow-
men.